HEALTH HELPERS

DOCTOR

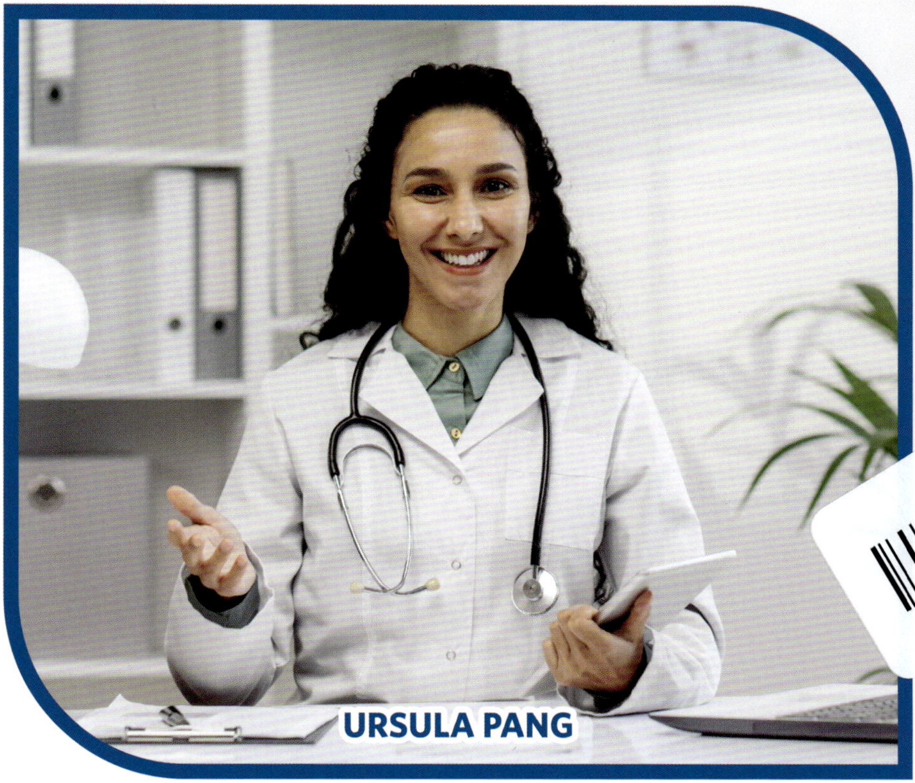

URSULA PANG

PowerKiDS press

Published in 2026 by The Rosen Publishing Group, Inc.
2544 Clinton Street, Buffalo, NY 14224

First Edition

Editor: Greg Roza
Book Design: Rachel Rising

Photo Credits: Cover, p. 1 voronaman/Shutterstock.com; pp. 4, 6, 8, 10, 12, 14, 16, 18, 20 TechSolution/Shutterstock.com; p. 5 Studio Romantic/Shutterstock.com; p. 7 Casper1774 Studio/Shutterstock.com; p. 9 fizkes/Shutterstock.com; p. 11 kelvn/Shutterstock.com; p. 13 stockpexel/Shutterstock.com; p. 15 FamVeld/Shutterstock.com; p. 17 Elena Babanova/Shutterstock.com; p. 19 KOTOIMAGES/Shutterstock.com; p. 21 SeventyFour/Shutterstock.com.

Names: Pang, Ursula.
Title: Doctor / Ursula Pang.
Description: Buffalo, New York : PowerKids Press, 2026. | Series: Health helpers | Includes glossary and index.
Identifiers: ISBN 9781499456493 (pbk.) | ISBN 9781499456509 (library bound) | ISBN 9781499456516 (ebook)
Subjects: LCSH: Physicians–Juvenile literature.
Classification: LCC R690.P36 2026 | DDC 610.695–dc23

Manufactured in China

CPSIA Compliance Information: Batch #QWPK26. For Further Information contact Rosen Publishing at 1-800-237-9932.

CONTENTS

Health Care Workers 4
Specialists 6
Your Family Doctor 8
Time for a Check-Up 10
Treating Illnesses 12
Treating Injuries 14
What Are X-Rays? 16
ER Doctors 18
Healthy for Life 20
Glossary 22
For More Information 23
Index 24

Health Care Workers

Doctors are highly trained health care workers. Most go to college for at least 8 years. Then they must work under other doctors before opening their own doctor's office. That's a lot of training! It makes doctors some of the most knowledgeable health helpers there are.

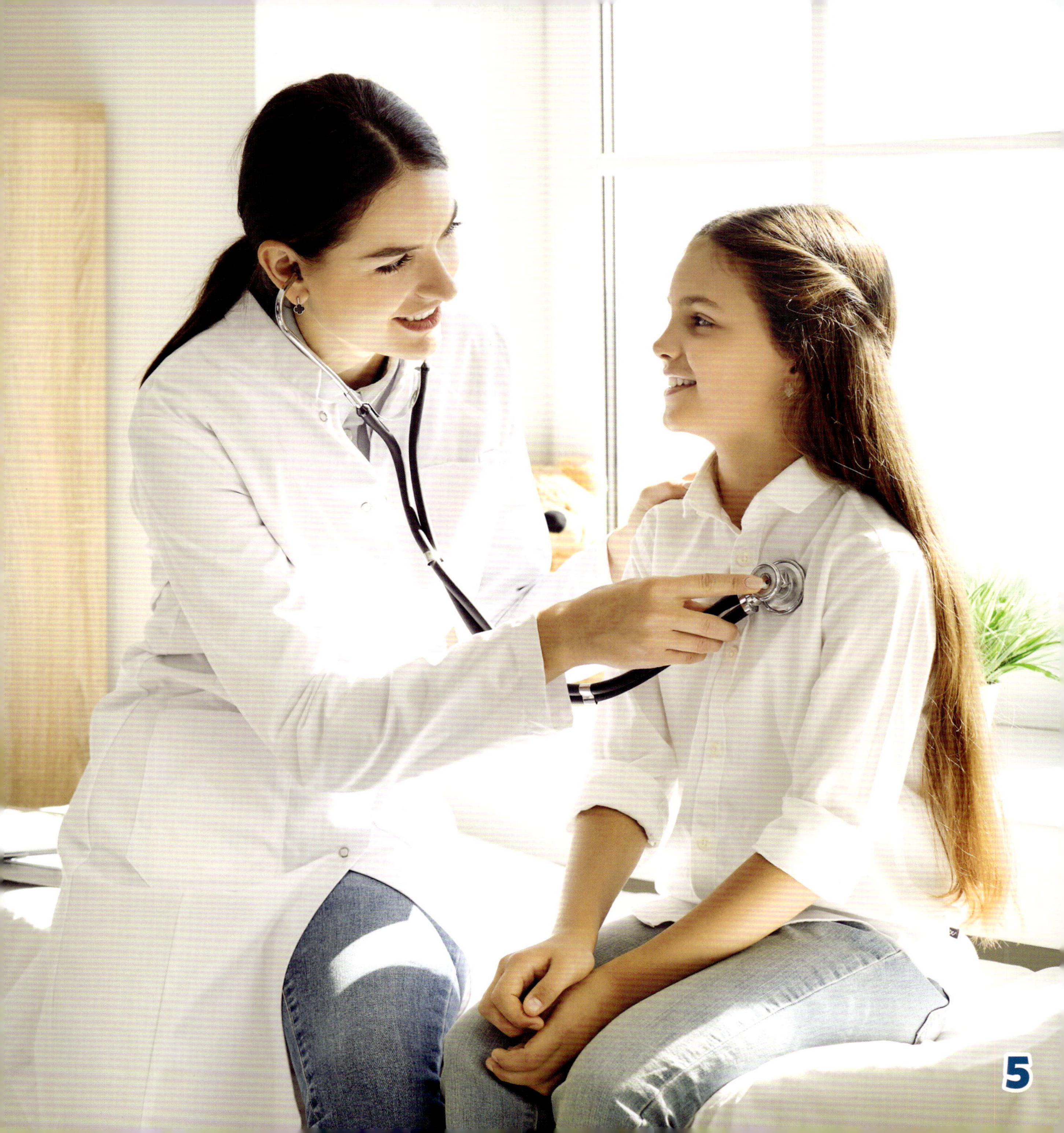

Specialists

There are many kinds of doctors. Some treat skin problems. Some treat eye problems. Some treat foot problems. There are many others! These kinds of doctors are called specialists. They become very knowledgeable about a subject, which makes them **experts** in that subject.

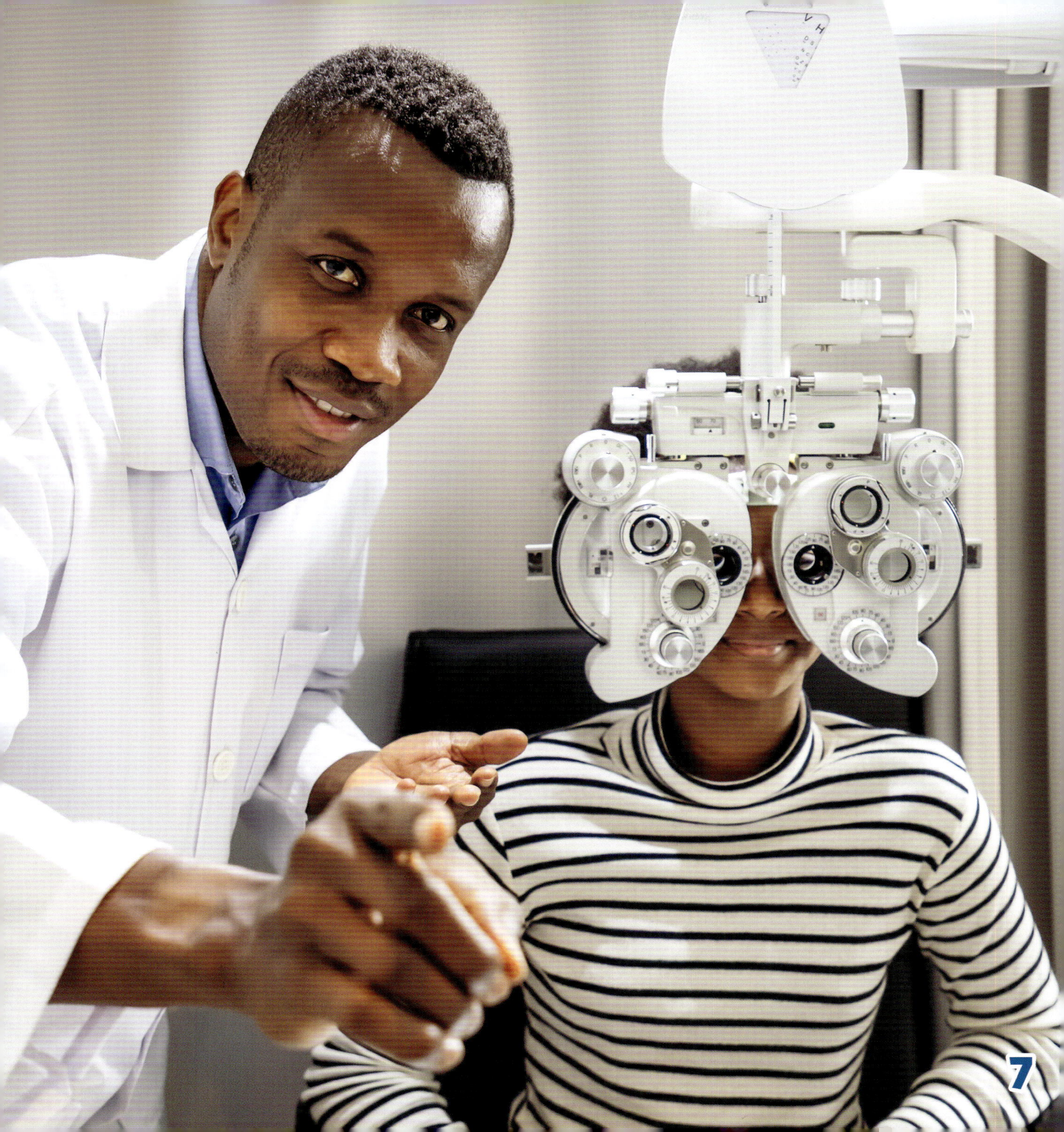

Your Family Doctor

Family doctors are called primary care doctors. "Primary" is another word for "first." They are the first kind of doctor we go to when we have an illness or **injury**. If a doctor discovers something they aren't trained to care for, they will send you to a specialist.

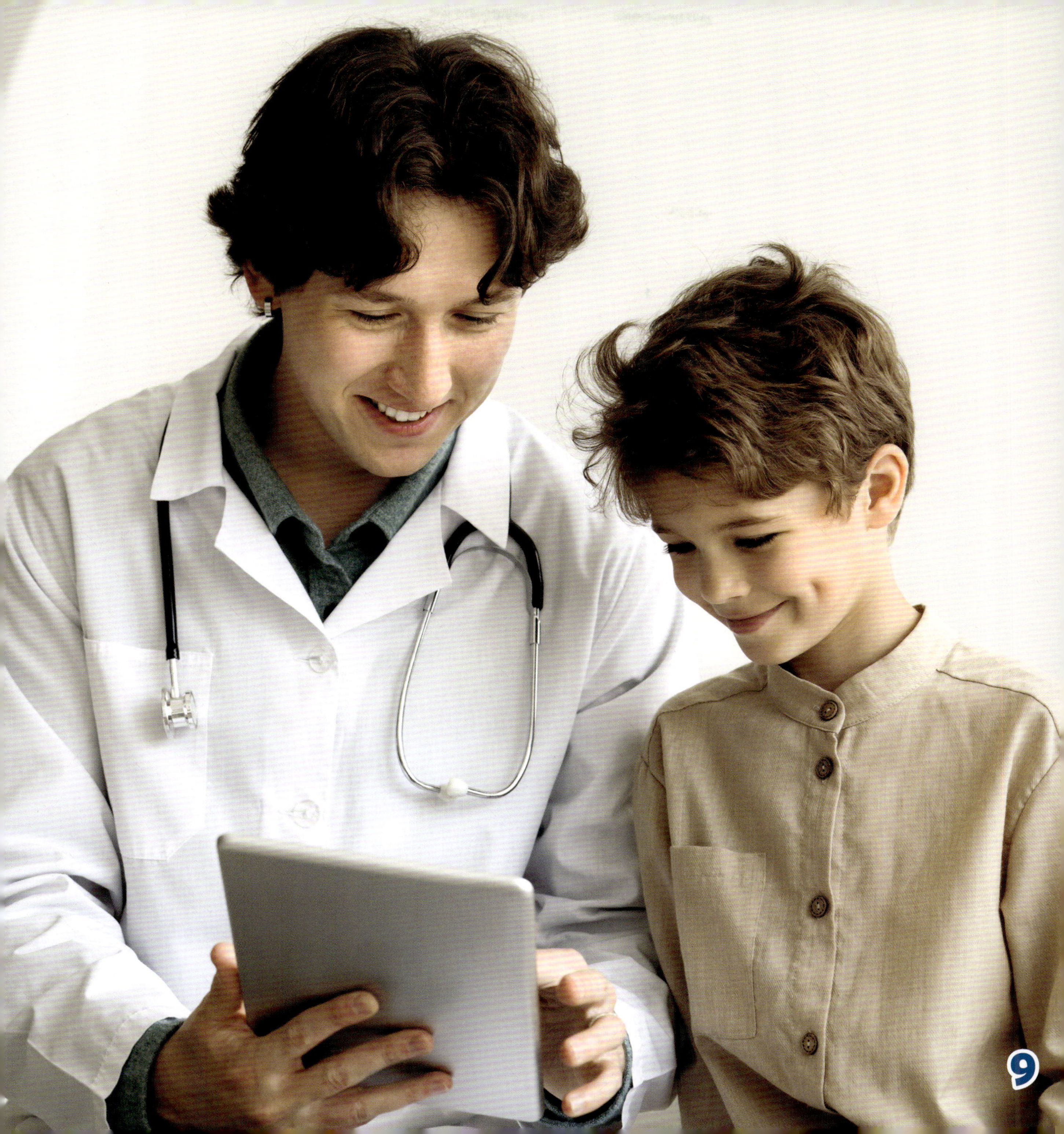

Time for a Check-Up

Most people go to see their family doctor once or twice a year for a check-up. The doctor will record your height and weight. They will listen to your heart. Doctors will ask you questions about your health. Doctors will also answer any questions you have.

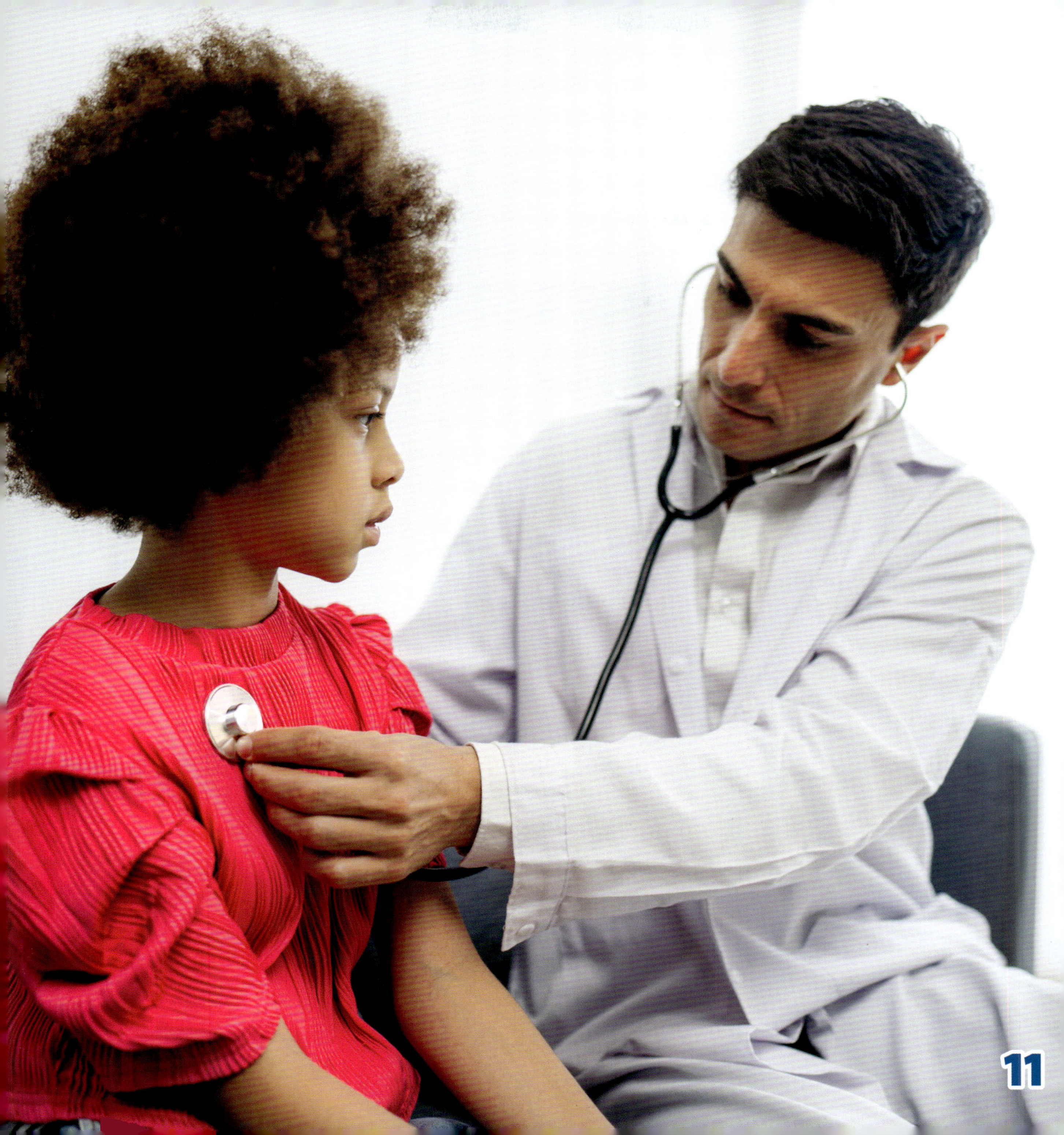

Treating Illnesses

You may go to the doctor when you are sick. You can make an **appointment** with the doctor. The doctor will use a **thermometer** to take your **temperature**. They will give you medicine to fight the illness. They might send you to a specialist.

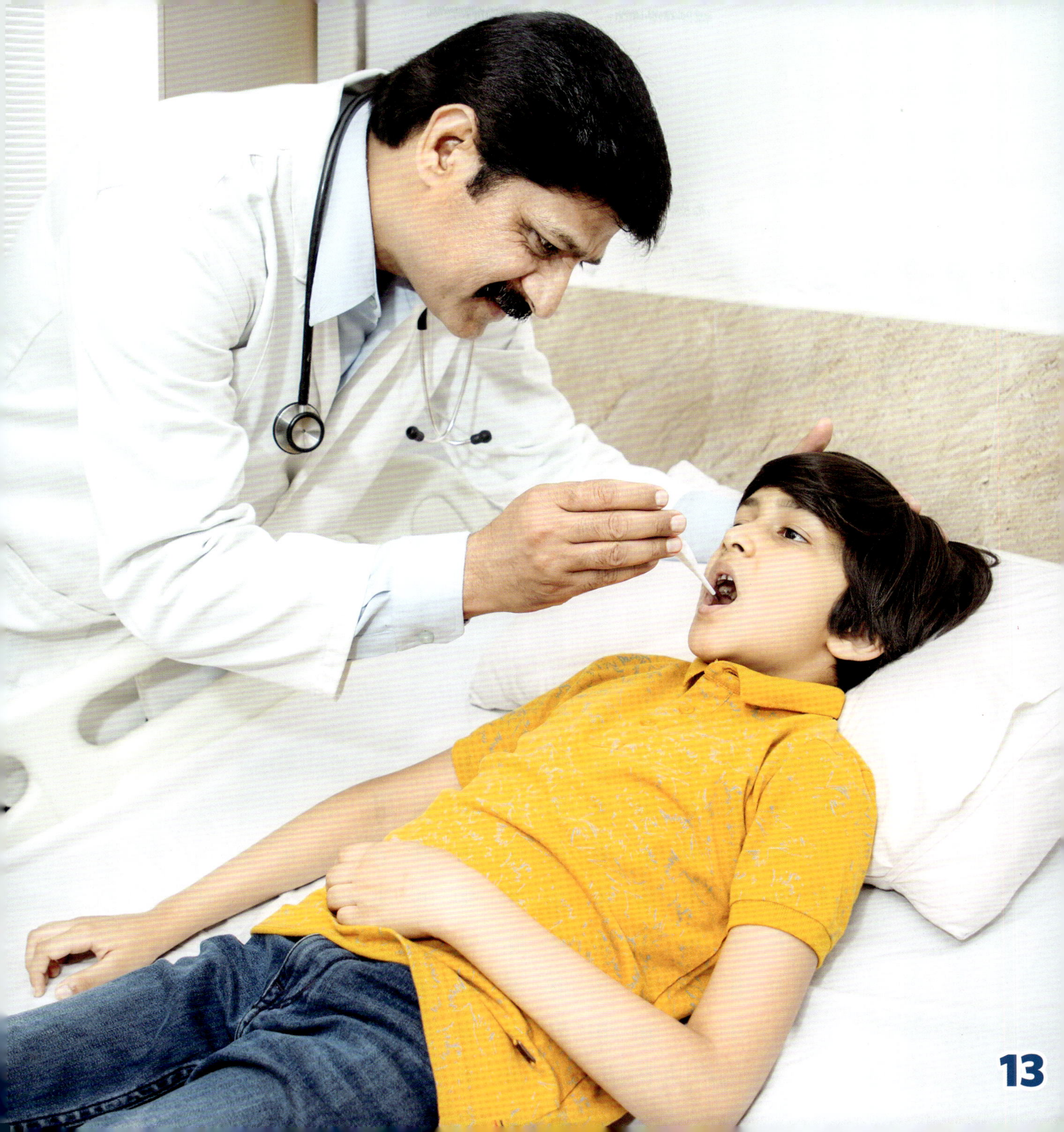

Treating Injuries

A doctor will give you a check-up if you are injured. Injuries can include burns, cuts, broken bones, and more. Injuries can be caused by **accidents**. They can happen when we are playing sports. Doctors may use an X-ray machine to look inside you!

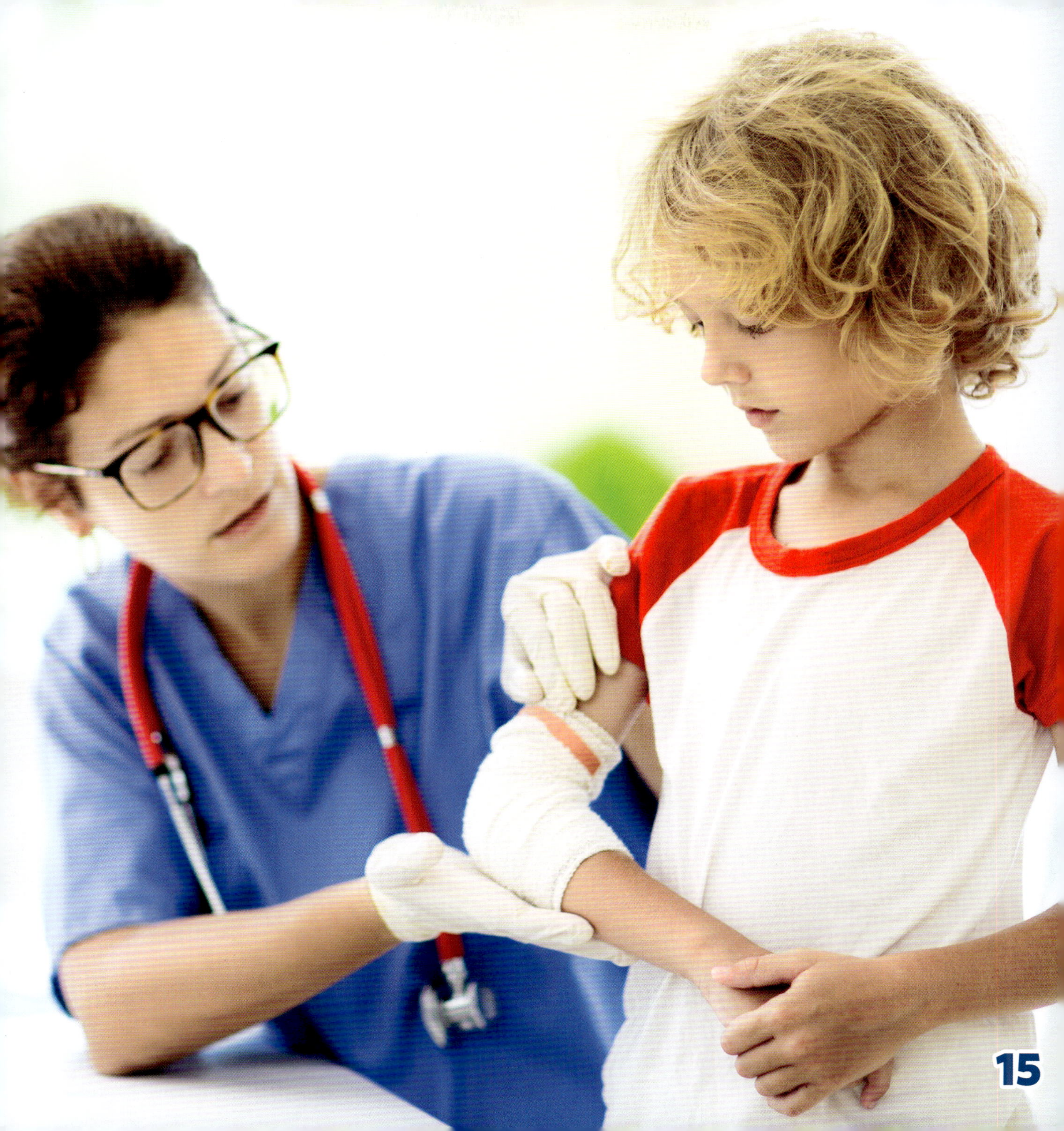

What Are X-rays?

An X-ray machine uses **radiation** to look inside the body. The machine makes a picture called an X-ray. Some parts of the body block X-rays. Bones block X-rays. That's why they show up in the picture. Doctors use X-ray machines to find illnesses and injuries inside the body.

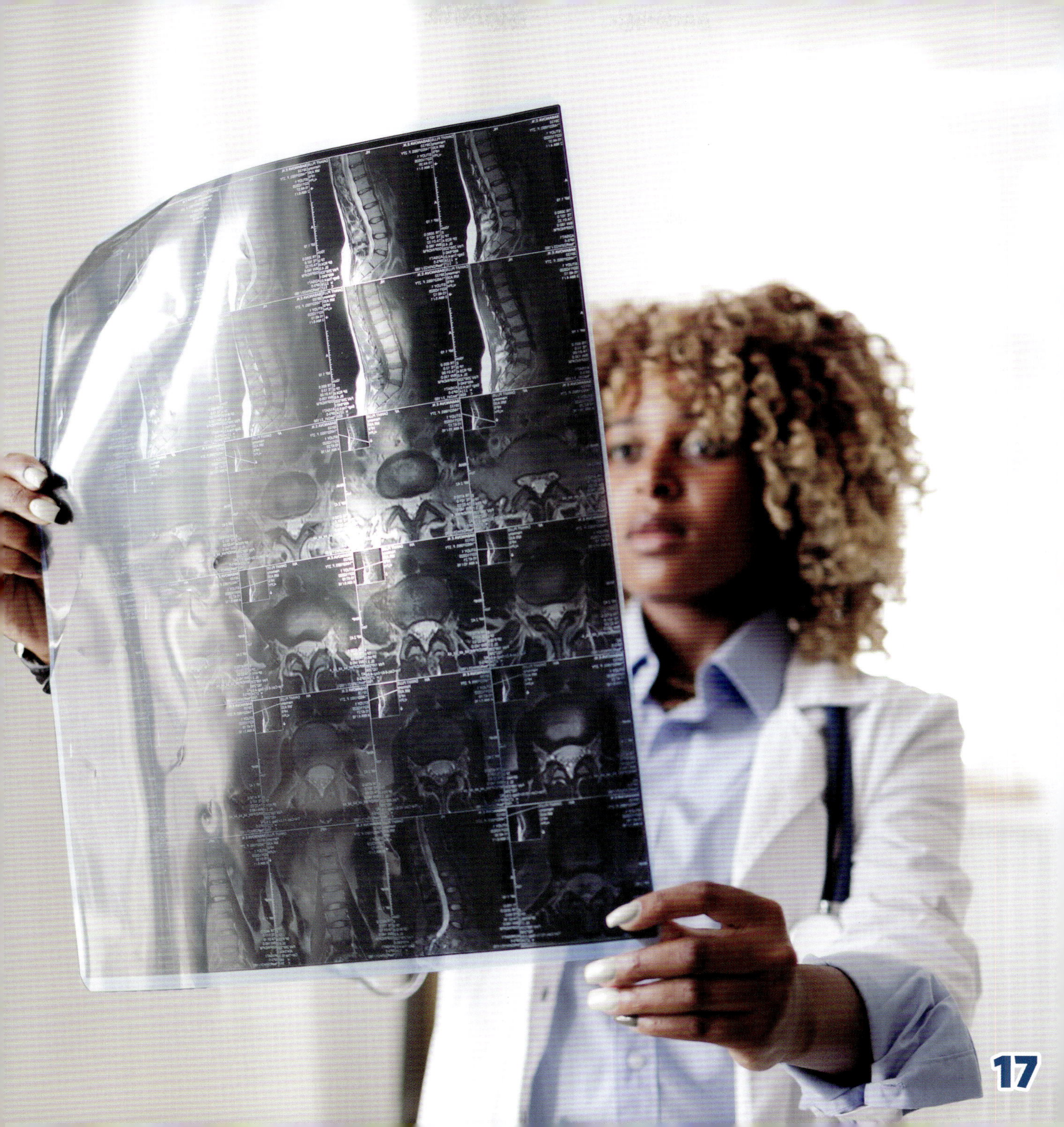

ER Doctors

Many doctors work in hospitals. The busiest place in a hospital is usually the **emergency** room, or ER. ER doctors often work many hours. They see all kinds of people with all kinds of illnesses and injuries. They are experts in helping people during emergencies.

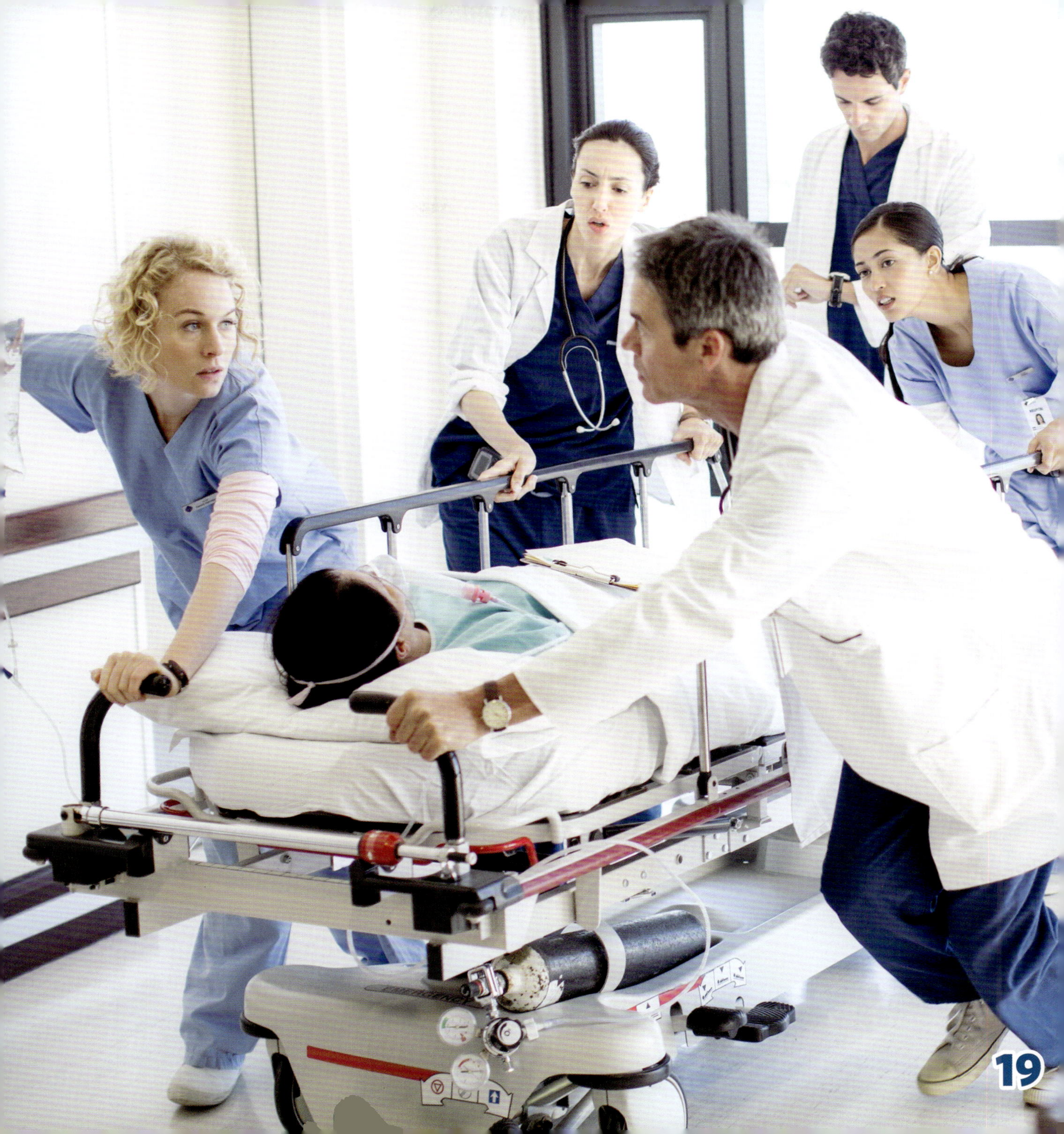

Healthy for Life

Right now, you probably go to a pediatrician. That's a doctor who treats people under 18. When you get older, you will go to a doctor who sees adults. Many people stay with the same doctor for many years because they like them and trust them.

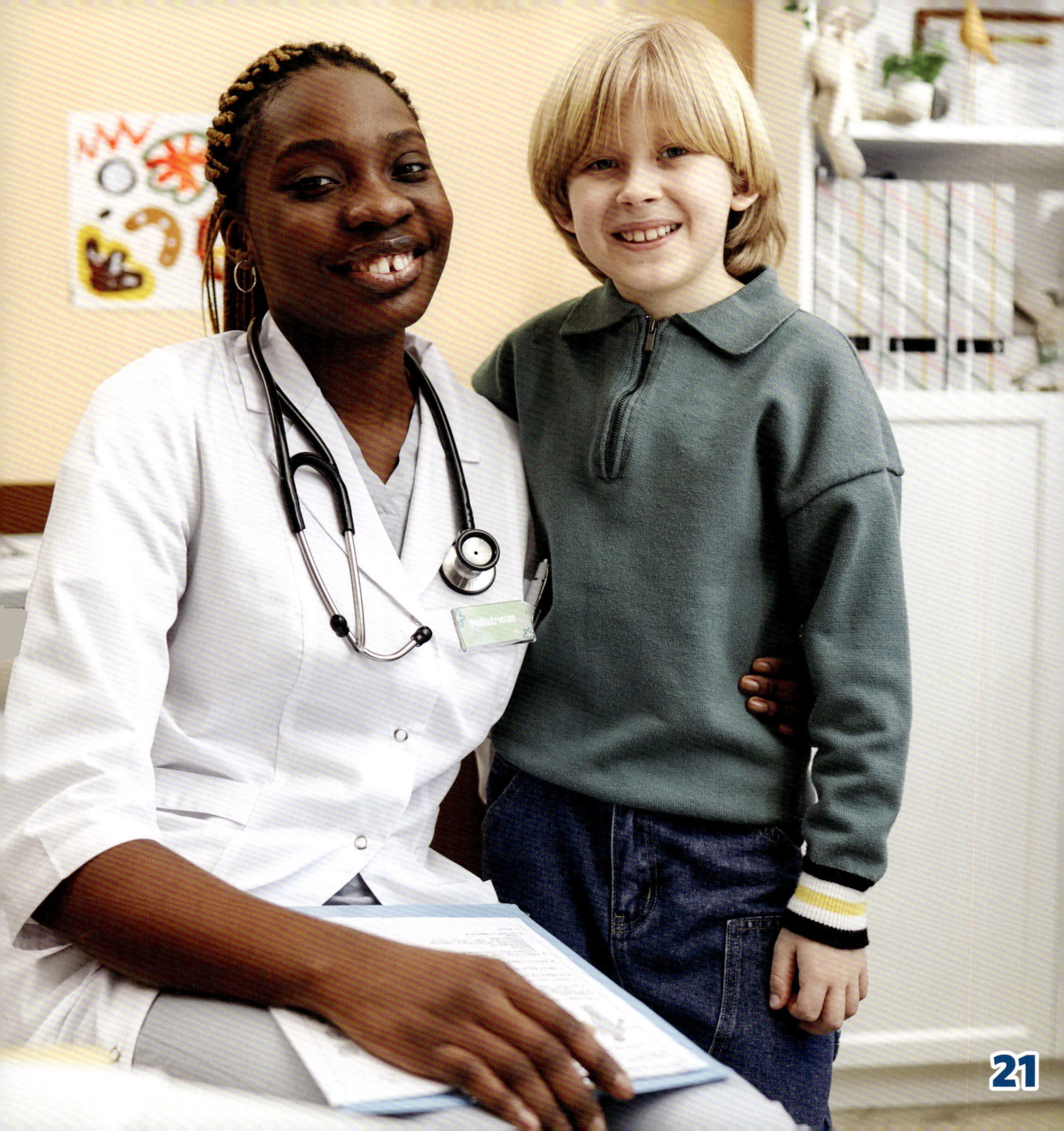
Pediatrician

GLOSSARY

accident: An unforeseen happening that is usually bad.

appointment: An agreement to meet at a given time.

emergency: A sudden event that calls for quick action.

expert: Someone who knows a great deal about something.

injury: Harm to the body.

radiation: Waves of energy.

temperature: How hot the body is. A higher temperature is a sign of illness.

thermometer: A tool that tells how hot or cold something is.

FOR MORE INFORMATION

BOOKS

Kukla, Lauren. *I'm a Doctor.* Rochester, MN: Mayo Clinic Press, 2024.

Lake, Theia. *ER Doctor*. Buffalo, NY: Gareth Stevens, 2024.

WEBSITES

Going to the Doctor
kidshealth.org/en/kids/going-to-dr.html?ref=search
Read more about doctors and why it's important to see them regularly.

Going to the Emergency Room
kidshealth.org/en/parents/emergency-room.html?ref=search
This webpage explains the A to Zs about the emergency room, from calling 911 to what happens after one leaves the ER.

INDEX

C
check-up, 10, 14

E
emergency room, 18
expert, 6, 18

F
family doctor, 8, 10

I
illness, 8, 12, 16, 18
injury, 8, 14, 16, 18

M
medicine, 12

P
pediatrician, 20

S
specialist, 6, 8, 12

X
X-rays, 14, 16